Fatgyrl purgatory

First and foremost, I am not a Dr. I am providing information that I have studied and natural remedies that I have been taught. Everything I speak of I have tested on myself. These changes have worked for me and I am sharing the information to benefit others. Do not stop taking your prescribed medicine if you are on any. Check with your doctor first before you start any routine. Acknowledge your ailments, allergies so you can incorporate healthy, long-lasting changes to eat yourself healthy!

We will be increasing water intake, water is essential and if you already drink a lot of water....drink more. Try to get to One 8 oz. glass every hour. If you think that's too much, it's really not because your colon uses water every half hour and you need to replenish it to help keep it functioning properly. Really. So until you are able to reach that goal try starting at 4oz. of water per hour.

Now this first week we will be training our minds and in turn taming our appetites. I am going to ask you not to really give up anything just yet, but to simply change when you eat it....really ☺ Sooooo the first week is just increasing water intake and addressing your health issues.

WHO AM I?

Glad you've asked. I am a mother, sister, friend and author ☺ I work a 8 to 5 job, I am currently studying to be a nutritionist, and I am one of the countless women that have been on every (and I do mean every) type of diet, taken every type of diet pill and bought every new exercise CD and still lost the weight loss battle. I *was* also overweight, suffering from depression, high blood pressure, acid reflux, and I was a borderline diabetic. I had come to a conclusion that fad diets (although they do work) and pills (no comment) were not going to be a permanent part of my life, so I got rid of them, all of them. I used to be in good health, we all were and then I started to experience some not so nice points in my life that derailed me from that path. I had an experienced a breakup that eventually lead to a divorce, my mother passed away and then my father, I lost my job that I was then employed for a number of years and I had 3 small children to take care of and wasn't receiving any financial assistance. (Whew, that's a lot!) It just felt like I hit rock bottom. And with that downward spiral, the weight came, and I didn't even notice or care and after a while I couldn't stop it. I let go of what I thought then was a healthy lifestyle and began eating everything in sight. MY NAME IS PURPLEBARBI, AND I AM AN EMOTIONAL EATER. Piling on the weight took its toll on my body, mind and spirit. It used to take me about a good 5-6 minutes to climb a flight of stairs, and when I got to the top, I was out of breath, my heart raced and I would be covered in sweat. I developed high blood pressure, acid reflux which resulted in having surgery to remove a piece of tissue in my throat due to the acid regurgitation, and I was becoming a diabetic. I was unhealthy *and* unhappy. When it was pointed out to me that I had high blood pressure, I was put on medication, I experienced side effects of one drug and was put on another, I developed low iron, and put on a medication for that and for those who take iron pills you know that wreaks havoc on your digestive system, so I was put on another medication to counter the effects of the iron pill and a pill for the reflux and I was going on another pill for diabetes. I wasn't even in my mid 30's! I was taking four different medications and I was miserable. One day I was walking into Wal-Mart (one of my second homes) and caught a glimpse of myself in the sliding doors, I didn't recognize myself, I had double everything, chin, belly, my arms and thighs looked like hams (which actually made me hungry at the time). I hadn't realized that I had let myself go… that far. I was like ……time for a change, so I said enough! I came to the point where it was time to take back control of my life, or that is what I told myself. I started working out and eating differently. I was working out every day and eating salads, vegetables, fruit and the weight stayed…yes, it asked me "Is that all you got?" It wasn't, I increased my workouts to twice a day, ate less and the weight stayed. I literally didn't lose one pound. So this went on for a couple of months and I gave up. I had a girlfriend that had high blood pressure and her doctor put her on the Tomato soup diet and she dropped a tremendous amount of weight and suggested it to me. I too lost weight about 25 pounds and when I finished that diet…… the weight returned. Going back and doing the same diet is impossible for me, so I tried another. I tried the Atkins diet. Yes, I was so excited to do this diet, because I was going to be able to eat all the meat, eggs and cheese and all the foods I was trying to deprive myself of. That lasted all of 3 days when I put on 6 pounds! Really ☺ There were many other diets, cleanses and pills. I have literally tried them all and the majority of them worked but after the time frame of the diet ended, so did my way of eating and I put back on the weight and sometimes more. I wasn't able to incorporate the diet into my way of living. I repeat, *I* wasn't able to incorporate the diet into my way of living, so something had to change.

CHANGING BARBI

After a few years of yo-yoing I came to accept my size and forced everyone else to do the same. I was a horrible person, I had a terrible attitude, and I was demanding, overbearing and just a plain asshole. I wanted more but didn't know how to because I was so miserable that it radiated from me like a repellant and ran off everyone that came within 10 feet of me. I looked mean, I talked harsh and even though I was efficient at my job, taking care of my kids, I really didn't have any relationships outside of that and the people that I did talk to were only at work or were in the same state of mind that I was in.....they were miserable too. So whenever I went home, I fed the kids and was done for the day and got prepared to do it all again the next day. I was in Fatgyrl purgatory.....and didn't even know it!

So I will flash back about 10 years before I got married, and not the marriage or whom I was married to were the problem. So anyhoo, I was younger, beautiful, and full of confidence and just all around happy or so I told myself. I had a great job, my own place, my own car and I did as I wanted, when I wanted. I had one child then and he wanted for nothing. I had all these things but I really wasn't happy, not really. I was longing for something, because even though things were going my way, I was still alone. I had an emptiness in me that I couldn't fill. I was in need something but I couldn't quite figure out what it was. Until recently. So once again we are 10 years back and I was fully committed to the dating scene and ended up meeting *him* and I eventually married *him*. So this was wonderful of course and I felt that it met all of my needs.

WARNING: Never think that another *person* will meet your needs, not even if you marry them. So that thought lasted all of 3 days, yes 3 days and I was like "Who the hell are you and where is that awesome guy that was just here…..literally 20 seconds ago! Ummm, excuse me where in the hell did he go?" That conversation is really how it happened, seriously. So instead of walking away, I stayed and spent the next 9 years looking for and waiting for the man I married to show back up, but he never came. And his doppelganger ending up walking out on me, leaving me with two children and pregnant with another with no help, any kind of help….smh. So there I was defeated or so I thought and after my last daughter was born, depression set in and the weight piled on relentlessly. The weight from being pregnant and then add on another 30 pounds of anxiety, bitterness and heartache on top of that. And yeah, you got about 180 lbs. of Barbi. Next my father had a stroke and was in need of care after that, and then my mother took ill and died suddenly! I was reeling, I didn't really have a good relationship with my mother but I loved her. I will always regret that we didn't *know* one another, everyone loved her but I knew nothing about her. After that there came another 20 or so pounds, and after countless reconciliations with my now x-him, more weight piled in on the fun and then my father died. I remember when he was at the point where he could no longer talk and when I came to visit him, he would lie in his hospital bed and just hold my hand and stare at me, I could see the love in his eyes. That was a blessing. So I ate and ate until I was full which put me to sleep. That put me out of my misery until I woke up and had to face my reality.

So let's jump back to the present, back to the sliding doors at Wal-Mart. I was walking in and caught a glimpse of 240 pounds of Barbi, I didn't recognize myself, I really didn't and needed to change. As I told you, I began working out, trying all kind of fad diets and pills and my weight loss was either temporary or minimal. I remembered when I was younger, I was fit, I lifted weights and ran almost every day and I decided to get back to that. I threw out all my medication (I don't recommend it) because it was just regulating my symptoms and not riding me of them. So I started drinking low calorie sodas, eating healthy cereals, diet meals and the weight was still stagnant and my symptoms worsen without my medication. I ended up going back on the meds and on my way to one of my appointments, a representative of the VA asked me if I would be interested in a nutrition class. I didn't have anything else to do so I agreed and am I glad I did. I was bored at first, talking about fruit and vegetables until the instructor pulled out a diagram of product labels. I had never before read the labels on anything I bought. Never and I was again in my mid 30's. So I then learned to consume more fruits and vegetable to lower my blood pressure naturally. So I tried that method. I wasn't a big vegetable eater, and the vegetables I grew up on consisted of corn, green beans, peas, cabbage, collard and mustard greens and I had Brussels sprouts once when I was younger as well. I had my first taste of broccoli when I in my 20's really☺. I used to eat fruit sparingly as well, and learned that it contained natural sugars, so I started eating more of them as well. You know how when you're younger and you how certain statements are burned into your memory. I remember a news segment on oranges and how eating about 4-5 oranges was like eating a cheeseburger, so I stopped eating oranges. So once again, I left this nutrition class believing that eating more fruit and vegetables would lower my blood pressure. So I again took myself off my medications and began buying and consuming more vegetables, and more fruit, and when I went out to eat I made sure to order a vegetable along with my meal. I eventually started to order just vegetables when I ate out, or just had a plate of vegetable for dinner when I cooked as well, but the weight loss was minimal and my blood pressure remained high and still had my other symptoms. So I gave up on that notion and went back on my meds. Another few years passed and I then tried the South Beach diet. It worked! And in about two weeks I lost at least 12 pounds, but I couldn't incorporate that diet into my lifestyle and the weight came back. So I continued yo-yoing on different diets and pills until I was up one night and watched an info-mercial on how a workout had changed this one woman's life. Her story was sad and I could relate to how being overweight put limitations on you and was encouraged to buy this product. Said product arrived and about after 2 weeks I stopped, because I did not see any results, yes the routine became easier to do but I was still overweight! Another fitness method came along and another and I would quit after 2 or 3 weeks and more and move on to the next new workout video that came onto the scene. I went from Tae-bo to the Firm (which I still have and use) and onto countless others. Even after all my attempts, the weight came back.

WHO'S TO BLAME

Now during all the years of weight loss and weight gain,
I was having issues. I was working, coming home taking
care of my kids, but I was a hermit. I didn't go *out*; I took
my kids to the movies or the mall every weekend. We
attended church, games, went shopping, to the beach...but
I didn't go out. I was always with or doing for my children,
and in the back of my mind I was waiting, waiting for my
life to change. My family seemed to have scattered to the
wind once my parents died and no one spoke to each
other (and rarely do today...) so I had no confidants to talk
to. So I waited, I was not admitting it to anyone but in the
back of my mind still waiting for *him* to come back (and he
did, and I took him back...as we all do and it didn't work as
it never does.) and I was angry when he came and angry
when he left. When I was up, I wanted to feel and look my
best, so I did and when I was down, I didn't care how I
looked and it showed. The weight came and went and I

eventually stopped taking or allowing pictures to be taken of me because when I saw them I saw my doubles and didn't want to accept that I was that far gone. So I just stopped trying to lose pounds and accepted that I was overweight and alone and would always be. In this time of acceptance, I met a young lady who was full of everything! She was beautiful and funny and she wanted to be *my* friend? She didn't seem to mind my weight and was like "let's go out for an afterhours cocktail, or "Come over for lunch" and the ultimate "Let's go out" I was ecstatic and concerned since I hadn't heard those words in years....from anyone. My friend introduced me to the Cooper River Bridge Run, I had lived in Charleston for over 10 years and had never heard of it...smh really☺ and this reintroduced me to running. I weighed over 200 pounds and ran that six miles in an hour and 20 minutes, which is actually good time. We became friends and workout buddies. I was getting in shape, losing weight, I was enjoying my new friendships and going to church and my kids and then......I met another him. It was good for a while but that too ended. That "end" took a toll on me and I stopped doing all the things I used to for a while and would then pick it back up and get back on track. So with all my loosing and winning, I still couldn't make a permanent change. So my friend saw some ladies running on the bridge and was intrigued by their shirts "Preserve the Sexy" really? So she informed me and wanted me to check them out, and I did and joined the most fabulous running group. Black Girls Run (do look them up) so I was running and working out, but still not losing the weight I thought I should. And then I met another *him* and as before was good and then also did not last long. Something was blocking *me*.

PUTTING IT TOGETHER

I used to work in a call center where your shift changed. I took a break at around 10:30 and would eat something and then another break around 1ish or so in which I would eat as well. My snacks would include something from the vending machine (i.e. cookies, candy bar, or chips) something quick. And then there was a change in all schedules and instead of taking breaks at 10:30 and 1ish, our first break changed to 11:15 and 2:30 ish. So when 10:30 came around I was in heat! I was hungry and I would shake and was irritable because I was used to eating at that time. But after about a week, this stopped as I adjusted to my new schedule. (Did you get that ….ADJUSTED to my new schedule) I had dropped some weight, not sure exactly how much because I had stopped weighing myself. I remember when my mother was in the hospital I weighed myself. The scale said 240 pounds and some ounces (this was the timeframe of my divorce, my parents passing and my overall lowest point in my life). I then determined that all scales were spawned from the devil and vowed never to weigh myself again. Anyhoo, I was running and exercising and eating what I thought was a balanced meal, and I went from a size 22 to an 18. And in the picture below I ran 12 miles that day. I'm the one on the far left. So once again I met another *him* and that as well ended, but I was *expecting* it too and it did....??

Anyhoo, I was driving into my second home after church and the message that day was "What are you thinking

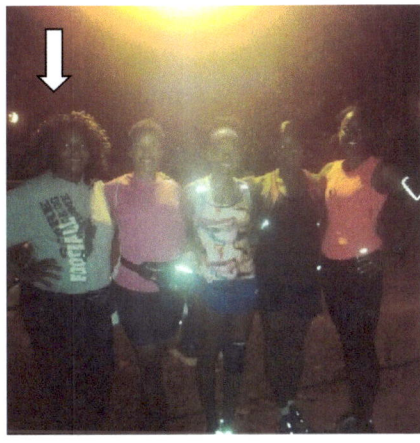

about?" or something to that effect. So my thoughts were angry, and I was always angry. And that was the message I received all day, from every channel I turned to, and every CD I listened to. Joyce Meyers said "Change your stinking thinking" Joel Osteen said "Control your thoughts" And I'm not sure how I heard or remembered (cause I don't) but had a little replay going on in my mind. "Change your thinking!" Trent Shelton, TD Jakes, Creflo Dollar...all with the same advice, what's on your mind. And when I really paid attention, I heard it? My mind talking...to me, reminding me of what happened when I was child, that my family was dysfunctional, how rude the cashier was when I went to the grocery store and that was about 7 months ago! How when I needed help and no one showed, but I was always helping others, and so on. Just stop for a second and you can hear your mind going off! Really! It took me awhile to get that under control and I'm still working at it, as long and you can create a thought you will have to monitor them. So in learning to take control of my thoughts, I learned to take control of myself and what and how I was doing things. I was so totally focused on the negative things that had already happened, that I wasn't realizing what was going on in my now. So some time passed and I thought I was working things in my favor and wrote a book about my past relationships and letting go of your past. "This is Your Vagina, The Vagina is Where the Heart Is" is the name of said book and I had the nerve to put it out there and watch what happened. Then I met another *him* and it ended and this time when it did I realized that I was doing the same things that I had written about in the book…smh. I asked myself "Isn't this what happened in the book?" And it was! Down to the letter **V**, and somehow I wasn't able to put two and two together and make everything in my life line up. One day, I was marketing my book and met a friend…Stormy (StormyWeather69) and by chance I was looking to get T-shirts made and she told about a movie to watch…"The Secret". So I watched it and gained some powerful insight, I looked up the speakers from the movie and was introduced to a whole spectrum that I didn't even know existed. Things began to change slowly, but change all the while. My last stop or intervention came from Shanel Cooper Sykes, a motivational speaker who literally helped me tie my spiritual lessons into my natural life. And I was like "okay?" because I could relate to her and understood what she was teaching. It took a couple of rounds with her for me to realize that *you* have to want the change and *believe* that *you* can achieve it! It all began with *me*, not with *him*, not *them*, not waiting on *God* or *miracles* but actively seeking and speaking the life *I* wanted into existence. And all this time I was just existing, not believing in myself not thinking that I deserved more, but I do and I did.

I began to "*speak*" to myself and not just let my mind steer me in whatever direction it wanted to and eventually I saw changes. I walked away from a few relationships, friendships and found "*myself*". I'm still working on self but I did in a different way, but from the inside out. Yes, I was and still a little consumed with what I and my surroundings look like, that's all I focused on. I had to have the right appearance and make everyone believe I was okay when I wasn't. And the first step was acceptance; I accepted my flaws and all the "*shit*" I had put myself through and allowing to happen to me. **(REPEAT: THAT I HAD ALLOWED TO HAPPEN)** Yes, where I was in my life was my own fault. It was a relief in a way that I now could stop blaming my ex, my ex friends, my co-workers, neighbors, the clerk at the store, the mailman (who was late sometimes) and whoever else decided to cross my path for my current status. I remember a commercial "Belly fat is not your fault" Really? Yes it is, and back fat and double chins all of that is your fault as it was mine. Would say I'm sorry….but I'm not.

FORGIVENESS

Is easier said than done. I don't know how many times I forgave the people who I *felt* had wronged me. The Bible says 7x77 times, I know I had come pretty close to that number. Anyhoo, I refocused and really started to pay attention to what I was learning in church. And in this span of 10 years I think I had attended every church in Charleston and Atlanta looking for a church home. God sent me an angel, Tonia Poteat, she was an awesome woman of God and I met her during an argument with my now x-husband. I was of course being myself and cursing him out about what I can't and don't try to remember when this little well-dressed lady walked past me and said "Stop all that" She sang. "It's a beautiful day and you're alive!" I'm so glad I held my tongue, because she became like a second mother to me. Thank you God for her. So I found a church home (Word Ministries, Summerville, SC) and felt welcomed, not pressured, at ease and I began to learn. Things didn't bother me as much anymore because I didn't focus on them, I dove into God's word and improved. God is still working on me.

So as my mind is being cleared and my spirits lifted, my weight was still the same. I broke my vow and weighed myself. I started to weight myself ever 3-4 months and my weight would fluctuate between 190ish to 180ish, for a few years. I was working out, running, eating better; I was even telling other people how to lose weight and once again threw out my medication and was determined to eat myself healthy. I was including vegetables for breakfast, lunch and dinner to get the required amount of nutrients in my diet. I was watching TV one night and came across a documentary on juicing called "Sick, Fat and Nearly Dead" it gave me a source of how to get the amount of nutrients and vitamins in my body without eating 12 cans of vegetables a day. So I tried juicing and it worked and was actually pretty good, this I could incorporate into my lifestyle and eventually did, and from there went on to smoothies and was introduced to all other kinds of living

that I was originally deemed for "people other than

myself".

CHANGES

Anyhoo, I was at a VA appointment and was again asked to attend a nutrition class, and I did and again was instructed on how more vegetables can reduce your blood pressure. Something about this was different, I was actually paying attention! When I attended before, I had so many other things on my mind that I all got out of the class was to eat more fruit and vegetables, and there was so much more. Same teacher, same set up but this time she brought an example of a can label.

"You need to read the label on everything you buy" She said. "Your salt intake should be less than 1200mg per day and watch the serving size of the cans you buy."

W-What? Cans had labels with information on the back of them? And it gave you the ingredients and serving size! How long has this been happening and why didn't anyone tell *me*? At the end of the class I had a thousand questions, and took the paperwork that was given.

"Why didn't you teach this in the last class?" I asked astonished by the new information I had received.

"I have taught this class for the past 3 years and have actually added more information to it" The instructor replied calmly. "And this has always been a part of it."

So it was me, I was the culprit and my mind (my Minnie Me) was the accomplice. After this course, I went home and reviewed what was in my cabinet, read every label and was having to eliminate a lot of things from my household. Canned foods, 320 mg of sodium per serving, boxed dinners 980 mg of sodium per serving, and my favorite...soups, 420 mg of sodium per serving and almost every item had 2 to 3 servings each. So I had to make a change and make it I did. Certain things I stopped buying and started cooking my own vegetables but still used Bar-b-que sauce, spaghetti sauce, mayonnaise, vegetable oil, still bought cookies , ice cream, still at fast foods and so on. It took me a while to learn about processed sugars, starches, insulin levels, carbohydrates and the effects that fast foods have on the body. I am still in the learning process and learning what, when, and how to prepare foods. It's no longer an ongoing struggle but an ongoing adventure. I have learned to change my eating desires, not habits, desires. When I was hungry, I craved what I was used to eating. I would run and get a burger or hot dog or something quick and satisfy that desire, and then go to the gym twice a day and be stumped as to why I wasn't losing weight. Things were finally falling into place. I had to change what I was putting into my body, everything! So I developed a plan, I remembered when my lunch breaks would change and so would my bodies craving to be fed, and I would run and get that candy, chips or something processed to satisfy my desire to eat. And when my break changed, I had no choice but not to feed my body until my new break time came around, which was about an hour later. My body screamed and kicked for something to eat, but there was nothing, I just couldn't leave my station and go get a snack, I would be disciplined. Yes disciplined, just like I would have to be disciplined about my job, I was going to have to be disciplined about my eating. I read about weight loss, a lot and the key thing is more water intake. Simple enough, I'll just start drinking more water. Not so simple, I didn't like water and rarely drank it. But somehow I was going to have to discipline myself to drink it. It took me about 3 days to drink my first 8 oz. glass of water. Really☺.

So I was drinking more water, my bowel movements started to change and be more frequent, my urine no longer had that peanutty smell, but I was still a fatgyrl. Okay what's the problem now? I still couldn't figure it out. So I kept reading, the effects of sugar on the body, good carbs vs. bad carbs and just continued to learn and slowly make the necessary changes. I've taken medical classes, and I'm studying to be a nutritionist and the learning has never stopped. Fast forward to now. I have always heard that it takes 2 weeks to break and habit and 30 days to form a new one, so I put it to the test. I drank more water, cut caffeine, starches, and sugars and still I did not have the weight loss I wanted. I had changed made changes to my diet before, but not the right ones. So I again stopped all that I was doing and made a plan. I read how much water I should have a day and started to apply it, and instead of trying to make changes immediately I made then gradually, allowing myself to adjust to one change and then make another, and another and then some more. For me gradual changes were the keys to permanent weight loss. I spoke with my elders and those with natural weight loss cures, and asked my friends from different cultures what their remedies were and read a many books on Vegetables and fruit and what each one benefited the body. I educated myself, and came up with change. A change that would help cut our all the processed foods, sugar, and salt. A change that would introduce healthy, natural fruits and vegetables that offered a natural cure for what your ailing body needed, and in the interim......weight loss. My goal for this change was not to lose weight, because I had tried everything and seemed to be spitting against the wind. My goal was to free myself of everything that ailed me and once I was healthy, I could then incorporate my healthy eating into my lifestyle and then watch all the other areas of my life line up, including weight loss. With this challenge you can break out of Fat Gryl purgatory within 28-30 days, by adding more water, natural remedies, consuming more fruit and vegetables, eliminating salt and sugars. And with this challenge it is done gradually and you will be able to incorporate these changes into your lifestyle. **Now**....let's begin

WEEK ONE, DAY ONE – Increase Water Intake

This challenge can begin on any day of the week, so start where you are now. There will changes made throughout the week, no drastic diet changes (not yet) ...but **EXPECT** them and they'll come quick. Breathe, relax you can do this. First we need to add more water to your routine, so the first thing is to add **ONE** 8oz. glass of water **per hour.** Yes, **one** glass of water per hour....all day. Yes you can do it and no it's not stupid. The change is simple but it will take some discipline on your part. So for the first few days you are simply increasing your water intake. (Did you catch that, yep....the first few days) You'll want to drink at least 8 oz. glass of water per hour; most people can't. So start with 4oz. At the beginning of every hour, have a 4-8oz. glass of water. Now since you'll be drinking water first thing in the morning, **breakfast is going to move back by one hour.** Yes, have that first glass of water and then the second hour another glass of water and then eat breakfast.

This is what your morning routine will look like:

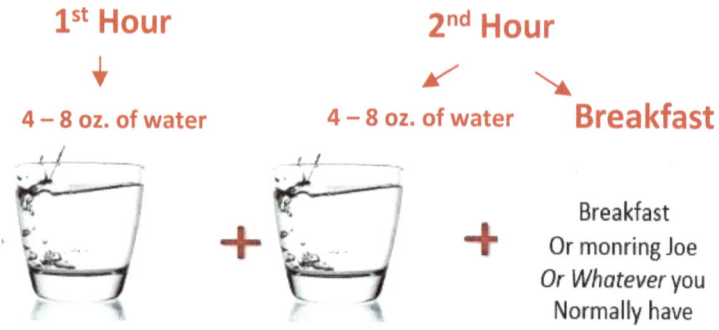

1st Hour

↓

4 – 8 oz. of water

2nd Hour

↙ ↘

4 – 8 oz. of water **Breakfast**

Breakfast
Or monring Joe
Or Whatever you
Normally have

Water is a major key to any lifestyle change or diet. Water hydrates your organs, promotes healthy digestion, flushes your system of toxins, and clears your skin, plus a host of other things. It takes less than a minute to make this change each day, so start drinking.

There will be changes every 3 to 4 days, they will appear quickly allowing your mind to get used to the first one, but not long enough for your body to resist. We are taking the body out of its comfort zone and giving it new instructions. While you're drinking you will need some ingredients for this week's changes. You will need a lemon, a bottle of Braggs Vinegar (with the mother), honey and of course water. This will be your "morning brew" gather your ingredients and be ready to start them on day *THREE*, this will replace your initial glass of water in the morning. , and remember to push breakfast back one hour. So on day three you will start your morning with the "brew", second hour will be another glass of water and then have breakfast. So if you were waking up with that morning cup of Joe or oatmeal, you can still have it just after you've had your brew and water. So you will be pushing any and all consumption besides "the brew" and water back by one hour… Trust me there is a method to the madness, promise and you have 3 days to ready yourself, so go and gather those ingredients. See ya in a few days☺.

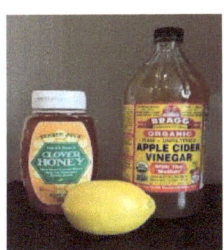

WEEK ONE, DAY THREE – ADDING THE "BREW"

We are still adding water, but today there will be an addition to the water intake. I specifically added this to my routine because I suffered from high blood pressure and acid reflux. This is a natural remedy that worked for both of my ailments and countless others and it has been tweaked time and time again. The first thing you will consume today will be "the brew" hope you've retrieved your ingredients as it's time to add to your routine.

Ingredients
3-4 tablespoons of Braggs Vinegar (with the mother)
2 tablespoons of Honey
1 squeezed lemon (not bottled)
One 8oz glass of water

Add all of your ingredients to your 8oz. glass of water, blend and drink. Some prefer "the brew" warm and served as a tea or even add a ½ tablespoon of cayenne pepper to kick start the metabolism or even ginger, there are many different ways to skin this cat. Now the brew is not that bad, really. And for some, if you don't like the taste, add another teaspoon of honey. Also, you may experience a little cramping as well, but it will subside. For persons suffering IBS, this will help and depending on the severity of your case, it may cause diarrhea, but allow your system to adjust to this change so it can work for you. Try halving all of the ingredients except for the 8oz glass of water. Now you have 3 days to get your changes in and under control. You can do this! Four weeks go by fast and week one is almost complete. So hang in there and get that water in!

The brew can be tweaked to serve you.

If you want to jumpstart the metabolism, add ½ tablespoon of cayenne pepper

If you have pain from inflammatory conditions such as osteoarthritis add a knuckle or 2 of fresh ginger **(grate or juice) to combat those symptoms. Ginger also decreases the risk of colon cancer, relieves nausea and vomiting, relieves the paid on dysmenorrhea (severe menstrual pain). Relieves symptoms of IBS, stimulates blood circulation and may prevent stomach ulcers.**

Turmeric can be added for joint pain as well. Add ½ tablespoon of Turmeric

Turmeric is a potent but safe Anti-Inflammatory spice. It can be used to treat flatulence, jaundice, menstrual pain, lower cholesterol, relieve chest pain, and pain from Rheumatoid Arthritis, Cystic Fibrosis, improves liver function and fights colon cancer.

Your day should be shaping up to look like this;
You've added your brew first thing (tweaked for your ailments) and consumption of food or anything else has been pushed back an hour.

1st Hour   **2nd Hour**

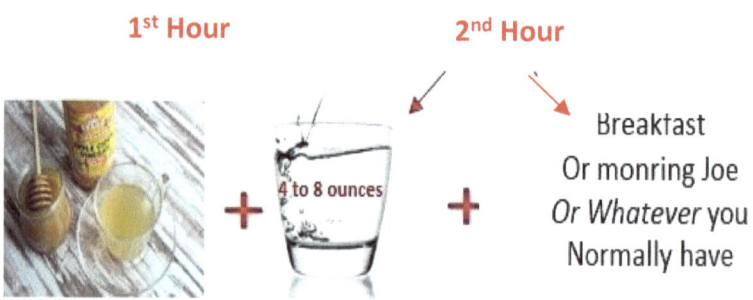

4 to 8 ounces

Breakfast
Or monring Joe
Or *Whatever* you
Normally have

Afterwards, continue with the 4-8 oz. of water per hour!

You are going to continue with your water intake and as I told you, there will be 3-4 changes each week. **Today**, we are getting rid of *added sugar*. I chose to start with sugar removal because that appears to be the hardest obstacle to overcome (it was for me). There is already sugar in everything; we are eliminating what you **add** to your meals and drinks daily. Added sugar has no nutritional value, it can damage your metabolism, cause diabetes and weight gain, So if you have packaged sugar, your neighbor is going to love you... pass it on. This includes sugar substitutes....even stevia.....rid yourselves of them. This will also include.....wait for it.....all carbonated drinks! WTF! **But not yet!** Calm down, relax, you can do this! I would say I'm sorry they have to go but I'm not. Sodas, energy drinks and other carbonated drinks and yes, even alcohols are loaded with fructose and sugars, and actually weaken your bones. "Your kidneys will thank you for their removal! In the meantime, try sweetening your drinks with honey or fruit. Once again you're not going to get rid of those carbonated drinks today.....you're going to rid them TOMORRWO! Yes, tomorrow and that doesn't mean run out and drink all of them that you can, it means get prepared for the removal.

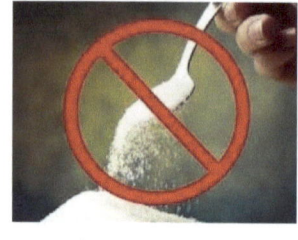 Starting right now, no more added sugar!

WEEK ONE DAY FIVE – NO CARBONATED/CAFFIENE/HIGH SUGAR CONTENT DRINKS

Hold the phone, yes and you are correct I said it…. no more carbonated drinks! No sodas, no energy drinks, no sugar free drinks, no juices, no sports drinks, no coffee and wait for it…….no alcohol. I would say I'm sorry, but your liver is screaming Hallelujah, really I can hear it from here. But the sugar in drinks is a main contributor to halted weight loss. The body can only process 4oz of nutrients from any drink, juice or what have you and then it's just straight sugar that you're consuming from there, really☺! This change is going to stabilize your blood sugar levels, prevent Psoriasis of the liver and improve its overall function and also allow all the water your drinking to flush your system as well. If I missed something from the no's, you still can't have it. So as of right now….yep, right now…

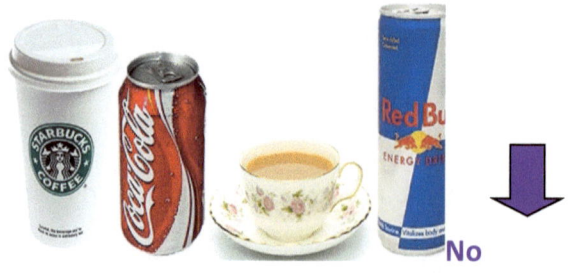

No

Carbonated/Caffeinated/ High Sugar drinks

CONTINUE WITH YOUR CHANGES THROUHT DAY 6; YOU WILL BE ADDING **GREEN** TEA TOMORROW, SO HAVE IT READY!!

WEEK ONE, DAY SEVEN: ADDING BACK A LITTLE CAFFIENE

As I said, you will be adding **Green** Tea to the mix. I know no caffeine, but this is a better caffeine and will calm your urge to binge on caffeine and sweets while burning fat. Yes, **Green** tea is a fat burner and will flux the toxins out of your system.   Add a cup of **Green** tea to your morning routine. Sweeten with honey or fruit like cranberries or raspberries, since you are not adding sugar.

So you routine will look like this: All food consumption is moved back as well

1st Hour   **2nd Hour**   **And then Breakfast**

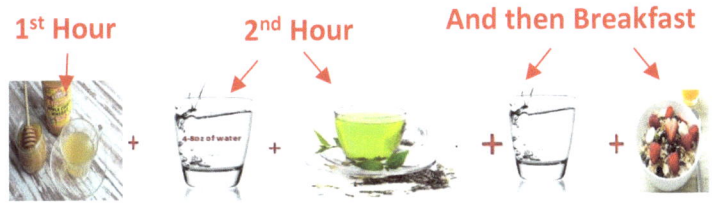

NOTE: The tea can also be tweaked to suit your needs, if you suffer from allergies, try peppermint tea, Dandelion tea if you have inflammation or need a diuretic, Chamomile to help regulate diabetes, or Hibiscus as it lowers high blood pressure. There are a many different teas for different symptoms. Investigate your symptoms and find a suitable tea for you.

WEEK TWO, DAY ONE- REMOVING ADDED SALT

If you have Table salt, sea salt, seasoning salt, garlic salt, onion salt, anything with the word salt on the end, even salt substitutes have to go. I would say sorry...but this change will be lower your blood pressure, save the body from osteoporosis, kidney stones, heart disease, organ failure, stroke and provide a host of other benefits. . So stop using that salt, take the shaker off the table, and give that container to a neighbor if you like but as of today

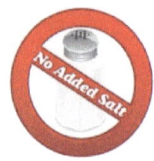 **No More Added Salt.**☺.

Assignment: I will give out assignments that have to do with upcoming changes for each week. As I said previously, salt and sugar is in everything. Hidden in the products we buy from peanut butter to bagged salads. Your task is to find it and be prepared to lower the amount

that you use or eliminate it all together (eliminate, that choice is up to you) but for now we are lowering your salt and sugar intake. You will have about 3 days before this change takes place so start getting prepared now. If you don't read labels like half of the country doesn't, let's begin. If you're at home or in a store or wherever you are, pick up a can or box or the granola bar, chips, etc. and turn it over. Yep, turn that bad boy over and look at the little box (Nutrition Facts Label) with all that information on it. It tells you every ingredient and serving size of your product. Right now we're focusing on sodium and sugar content. The recommended amount of salt consumption is less than 1500mg of sodium a day, or just a little over a ½ tablespoon of salt.

- 1/4 teaspoon salt = 575 mg sodium
- 1/2 teaspoon salt = 1,150 mg sodium
- 3/4 teaspoon salt = 1,725 mg sodium
- 1 teaspoon salt = 2,300 mg sodium

There *is* a difference between salt and sodium...yes. Salt is made up of 40% sodium and 60% chloride; it's natural and you actually can't live without it. Sodium helps you maintain your blood's water content and balances the acids and bases in the blood and moves electrical charges in the nerves that move our muscles. It's the inability to remove the sodium from the body that increases high blood pressure. And sodium is in everything, especially processed foods. Canned meats, vegetables, cold cuts, sauces, cheese, pickles, and sodas to salad dressings. Just about everything has sodium; even the salt substitutes contain sodium. The salt shaker is not where the majority of sodium comes from; it's from these processed foods that I mention. It's hard to lower your sodium intake, especially if you don't know how much has already been added to your product. Reading your labels is **very** important. Sugar is equally hard to control if you don't know what you're looking for. The same for salt read your labels and check you sugar content. While with **sugar** you want to have the amount per serving between **10-15 g** and no more than 25 gm per day for women and 37.5 gm per day for men. If you're diabetic, you want less than that and **do not** want to consume sugar daily. Another thing to watch for when controlling your sugar intake is HFC or High Fructose Corn Syrup, HFC is a sweetener used mainly in sodas and other flavored drinks and has found its way into almost every packed product on the market. This sweetener boosts your risk for diabetes, heart disease and weight gain. When you read your labels if you see items that have "tose" or "ose" at the end of an ingredient, leave it on the shelf.

READ YOUR LABELS!

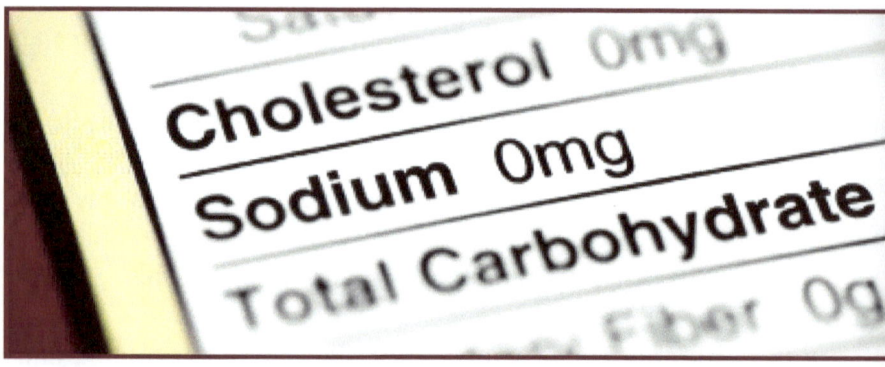

Get used to reading the label for everything you buy from this point on, this will take time but do your best. Once again you have a few days. We would like our labels to read 0% sodium, but most of them won't so your goal is to try and have 180-200 mg of sodium or less per serving of any product you buy. Those labels not only tell you how much sodium in your product, but how much sodium per serving. Really☺ You will be amazed the amount of sodium per serving per product you were consuming. I know I was. So once again learn how to read those labels!

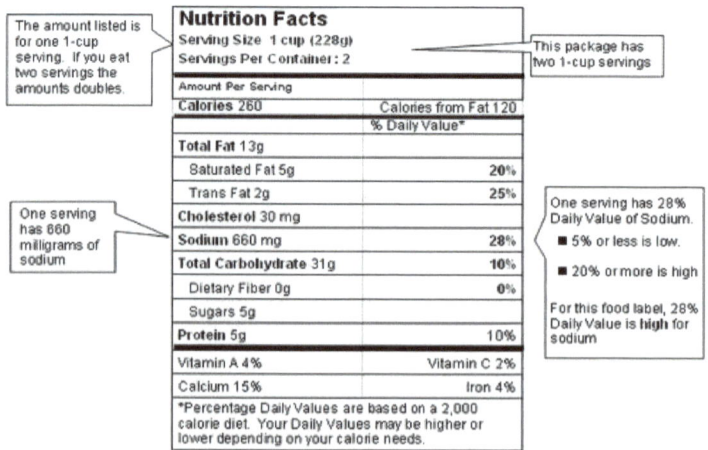

WEEK 2, DAY TWO – LOWERING SODIUM AND SUGAR INTAKE

As I promised, the day has arrived for you to stop the sodium and sugar. You are already removing added salt and sugar (What you actually add to your food) So no you're going to remove the hidden sodium and sugars that in food that are already packaged. Hopefully you were good pupils and have been reading your labels over the past few days, astonishing yes? All that sodium in a boxed meal or in soup for that matter. Sodium is in everything, even fresh vegetables so there is not a way to eliminate it, but there is a way to lower it so that it doesn't harm you. So continuing with your week one changes and now lowering that sodium. Now if you read the labels of your products, it should have 180- 200 mg of sodium per serving and remember you are not trying to exceed 1500 mg per day. You will also need to keep track of your sodium intake. Write it down in a food journal or a notebook, something you will keep up with or better idea, create an

Excel Spreadsheet that works great as well. Sugar intake you want to have no more that 10-15 gm of sugar per serving in your products, no more than **25 gm per day for women and 37.5 gm per day for men.**

WORKOUTS

As promised there would not be any workout until about week 3, so you are going to get your bodies ready to start. You're already drinking water to hydrate your muscles and get your blood circulating; now you will start stretching. As I said no need to run and buy those cute workout clothes (right now). So what you're going to add is just simple stretches as for next week you will start an actual workout.

Relax, you'll be able to handle this and it starts you **TOMORROW**. (If you already have a workout routine, stick to it!)

Simple stretches for you

Bend at the waist and touch your toes with your fingertips. If you're not able to do so go as far as you can (Hold for about **30** seconds)

Next: Stand straight with your right hand raised in front of you as if you're stopping traffic (so stop that traffic, stop it in the name of Love) and turn to the left. (Hold for about **30** seconds)

Next: Return to your standing position and do the same with the left arm. Raise it in front of you (stop that traffic) and turn to the right. (Hold for about **30** seconds)

Raise your left arm straight up and lean to the right. (Hold for **30** seconds)

Do the same with your right, lift that arm straight up and lean to the left. (Hold for **30** seconds)

These moves will take no more than 3 minutes to do, and that's all you have to do (for now).

So rest now and be prepared to add these stretches to TOMORROW'S morning routine!

Breakfast. We're going to change up breakfast. You will want to have a breakfast that includes no more than 200-400 gm of salt for the meal and no more that 10-15 gm of sugar. Now you have a lot to choose from. You can have fruit? ½ apple, ½ pear and a ½ banana will cover part of your breakfast. And you can add a slice of whole grain bread with a teaspoon of peanut butter. Also you can have a serving of steel oats (less sugar) with hazelnuts flaxseeds and almonds or an omelet with 2 eggs, spinach, onions, tomatoes, mushrooms and even low fat cheese. There are a thousand and one ways to fit 200-400 mg of salt and 10 - 15 grams of sugar into breakfast.

So for week 2, we're changing breakfast not to a specific thing but with a specific requirement of added sodium and sugars!

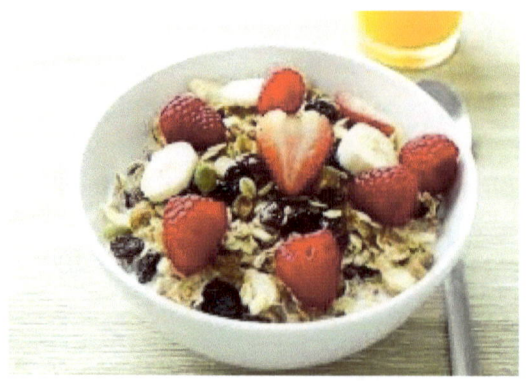

With the changes being made you should start to see a difference in your body. Your urine should be lighter and your bowel movements should be more frequent and a lighter color as well. You appetite should be different as well. Continue with your water intake as you will have one more change for week two. With all the removal of specifics from your routine, try some healthy alternatives. Instead of seasoning your dishes with salt, try different spices and vegetables do liven them up. Season your dishes with cayenne pepper, garlic, peppers, or even onions. Familiarize yourself with different spices that are beneficial to whatever ailment you may be experiencing. Try adding Turmeric, Cumin, Ginger, Cloves, Coriander, Sage and nutmeg to name a few.

For the remainder of the week you will be constantly, vigorously reading the labels of every product you currently have and purchase to lower the sodium and sugar intake of your routine. Also getting used to all the changes for the past and current week.

Week 3 starts in a couple days, and you will be adding more vegetables and fruit to your routine. Keep up your water intake, One 4- 8oz glass of water per hour!

WATER CONSUMPTION

Water is essential to your body function and it doesn't have to be bland. There are all kinds and flavors of water for you to consume. Remember you are eliminated all carbonated drinks, so that fizzy water is not allowed. Coconut water is an option, it has less calories and sodium that sports drinks and comes in different flavors. Aloe Vera water is a good choice as well. Aloe Vera water has anti-inflammatory agents and detoxifies bowels and helps absorption of minerals and it tastes good! Another alternative is to fuse your water. Yes water infusion, you are simply adding fruit to your water (specific fruit and mixtures of fruit) this is a great idea for diabetics who don't need to consume certain amount of sugars daily. Investigate the benefits of fruit and add them to your water!

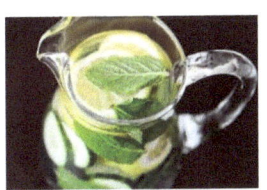

Lemon, Mint and Cucumber

This mixture is a great detox, the lemon helps cleanse and alkalize the body and boost the digestion and immune system.
Mint settles the stomach and aids in digestion
Cucumber rehydrates the body and has anti-inflammatory properties.
Ingredients
1 lemon (sliced)
1 large cucumber (sliced)
10 mint leaves

Add ingredients to a pitcher of water and allow to chill

overnight and drink for a quick cleanse.

WEEK TWO, DAY FOUR – NO MORE FAST FOODS

Yes, did I not mention that this was coming? I think I did

(remember, no drastic food changes as of yet?) Well if not

the day is upon us that we stop consuming fast foods! Yes,

no more burgers, tacos, burritos, breakfast croissants,

subs, pizza and the list goes on. So basically, if you buy it

pre-made, pre-packaged (this includes sandwich meats) is

now off limits! So as of now……No more fast foods! ☺

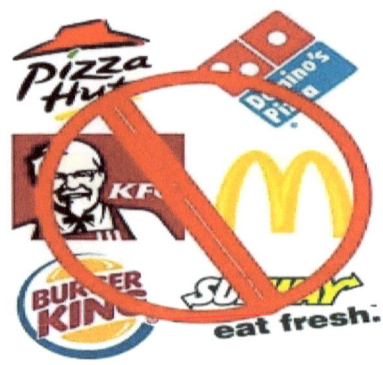

Note: Now that you will be preparing more of your own
food, watch what you cook with. Find healthy oils to use,
like olive or coconut oil (there are many). Breads are
becoming off limits but not all. You're able to have
breads such as Rye or whole grain which is harder for the
digestive system to process as it doesn't turn it quickly to
sugar. There are healthy substitutes for rice and pasta as
well, Quinoa, wheat or whole grain pastas. Investigate
and find a suitable one for you.

WEEK TWO, DAY 6 – ADD A GREEN VEGETABLE

Starting today, you will be adding vegetables to your routine and it will be added to dinner. Yes, dinner and ......and wait for it.... it must be green. Yes and why green? Well green vegetables are the most nutritious... really☺ Green Vegetables are good sources of Vitamins C, E, K, B2, B6, calcium, potassium, folic acid, copper, protein and iron. Now, I normally say that salad isn't a vegetable, but you can incorporate this in if you choose a salad for dinner. Choose a salad including kale, romaine lettuce or spinach would suffice; try not to use iceberg lettuce...no nutritional value there. Otherwise you have a host of other greens to choose from. Collards, Swiss chard, Turnips, Asparagus, Mustard Greens, Broccoli, Green beans, Peas and the list goes on ....for a while. So as of today you are adding a green vegetable to your dinner. ☺

WEEK 3, DAY ONE – NO DAIRY?

Yes no dairy! I'm not hearing any party in the background over there......Anyhoo, as of today, no more dairy. No milk, no cheese, no yogurt, and no nothing that contains dairy....bread as well you ask? Yes even bread ☹ The good thing is you don't have to give it to your neighbor because it should last for the next week or so and you can add it back after the challenge (if you choose) but in the mean time you will see that belly decrease, less gas and bloating. So starting today.....yes right now

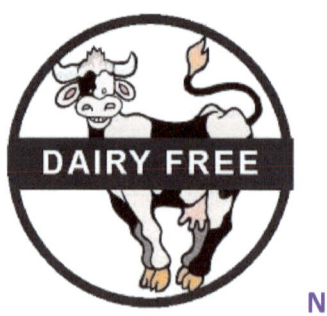

NO DAIRY

Yes this is the week you start adding exercises to your routine, if you already have a routine, stick to it. If not add these steps to your routine.

MAKE SURE YOU STRETCH BEFORE AND AFTER

Push Ups

You are only adding 10-15 of each to your routine. (Trust me it will be enough)

- If you're at the point where you can do 10 regular pushups, do them

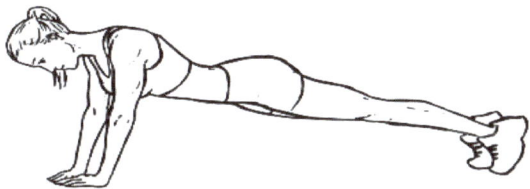

- If you need to do them on your knees, a push up is still a pushup….do them that way

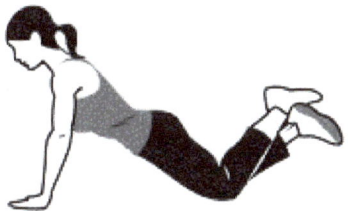

- If you can't get down on the ground, find a wall nearest you, lay your hands (palms flat) against the wall and take about 2-3 steps backwards so that you're at an angle and push from there.

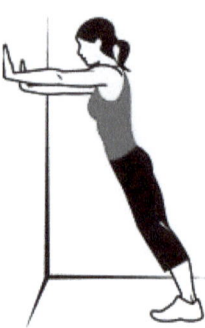

- Can't lean against the wall… place your hands together as if you are praying and press them together, hold that pressure for 10-15 seconds and repeat 10-15 times. You can do this!

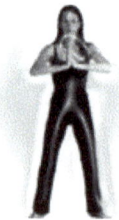

And you're done; you will be adding an additional exercise for the next few days

WEEK THREE, DAY TWO – ADDING MORE VEGETABLES

Starting today, you will be adding more vegetables to your routine and it will replace your LUNCH. Yes, replace your lunch, not added to it but replace it and ……and wait for it…. it must be green. Yes and why green? Well like before green vegetables are the most nutritious and since we've stopped dairy for now green vegetables will be your best source of calcium, magnesium and potassium.

So as of today you are adding vegetables are replacing your lunch!☺

NOTE: MAKE SURE YOU DON'T EAT THE SAME GREEN VEGETABLES EACH DAY, CHANGE THEM UP! COLLARDS ONE DAY ASPARAGUS THE NEXT OR HAVE 2 OR 3 DIFFERENT ONES PER DAY. ☺
NOTE: Make sure you get your stretches in! And keep up your water intake! In a couple of more days (two) you will be having a vegetable day, that's eating vegetables all day! For every meal! And they do not have to be Green. All day, as much as you want! Get prepared!

WEEK THREE, DAY THREE

Workout

Crunches – you will be adding 20 crunches to your routine, yes just 20 (now if you already have a regular workout routine, stick to it) trust me it will be enough. So lie down, knees bent at a 90 degree angle and pull yourself off the floor lifting your shoulder up and then return.

If you're not able to lie on the floor, do a standing crunch, it is just as effective.

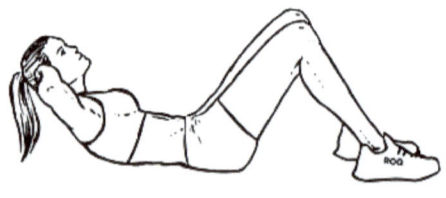

WEEK THREE, DAY FOUR – ADDING MORE VEGETABLES

Today you will be adding more vegetables to your routine.

Yes, you can't really get enough!   Today and all day you

will be having vegetables, that's right for breakfast, lunch

and dinner! And guess what, they don't have to be green!

You can have as much as you want all day.

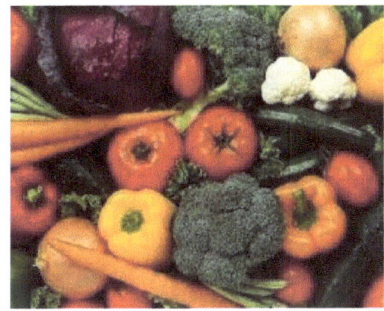

Don't forget to keep up your "brew", water intake, and

week 1 and 2 changes.

Continue with weeks 1 and 2 and your current changes. By the end of week 3 you should be down 10-15 pounds and better able to control your appetite. The only things you will be adding are more exercises.

SQUATS

A simple routine that will help strengthen your legs. Standing up tall, push your rear back as if you're about to sit down in a chair behind you. You're going to change your mind right before your bottom makes contact with the chair and return to a standing position. And that is a squat, now add 15 to your routine!

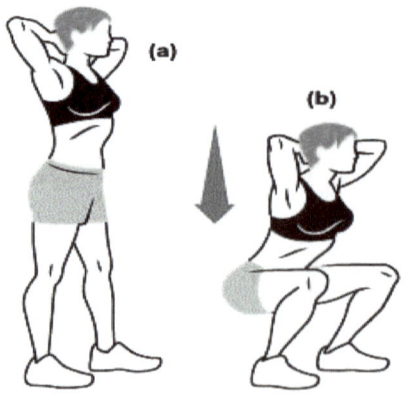

Four weeks goes by fast! You have one change this week and .....Wait for it...did the picture give it away? Yep, no meats. I waited to take away the good stuff till the very end. Yes even fish, is off the menu, but this is the last week! This is the home stretch baby so it's time to get it on! Once again you should be down between 10-15 pounds and this last week reach for another 5 pounds! You can do this. You will continue with your weeks One, Two and Three changes on top of week Four's addition. This week add on to your work out add more push-ups, crunches and squats as from here you will be to. Add another round of your stretches and workouts to your routine. You're stronger and healthier and these changes you will be able to incorporate into your lifestyle.

Following the plan will have allowed you to control your appetite, regulate your blood pressure, and stabilize your blood sugars and cholesterol levels. You should have a control on stomach irregularity. Now is the time to have your numbers checked and celebrate your success! With the challenge I created. I was able to rid myself of high blood pressure, acid reflux, regulate my blood sugar levels so that I was never a full blown diabetic and control my iron levels. I was able to eat myself healthy and the weight loss was an added bonus......in this process I dropped 20 pounds. I have implemented groups and some that join are successful and some aren't but all that stayed the course lost between 10-18 pounds and were able rid themselves naturally of their ailments like high blood sugar, high cholesterol, and IBS. I now have a plan that I can incorporate into my lifestyle and keep the ending results! I hope that the plan has provided you the same opportunity!

Please feel free to stop by my Facebook Page PurpleBarbi

30 Lifestyle Challenge for live participation.   Blessings!!!

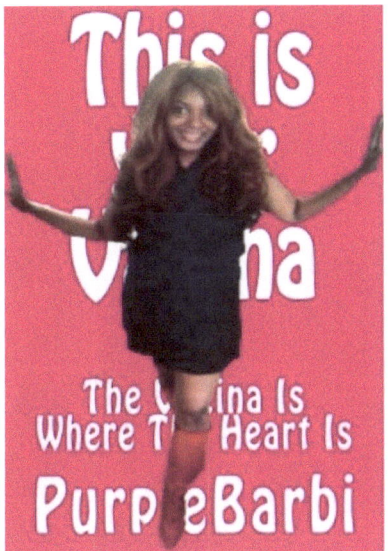

☺

www.ingramcontent.com/pod-product-compliance
Lightning Source LLC
Chambersburg PA
CBHW050813290526
45792CB00001B/96